Staff Manual for Adolescent Substance Abuse Intervention Workbook

Taking a First Step

Steven L. Jaffe, M.D.

Professor of Psychiatry
Emory University School of Medicine
Clinical Professor of Psychiatry
Morehouse School of Medicine
Atlanta, Georgia

Illustrations by
Darlene Berry Lauth

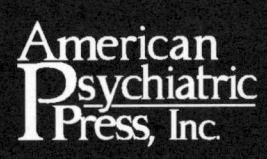

Washington, DC
London, England

Note. Books published by the American Psychiatric Press, Inc., represent the views and opinions of the individual authors and do not necessarily represent the policies and opinions of the Press or the American Psychiatric Association.

Copyright © 2001 American Psychiatric Press, Inc.
ALL RIGHTS RESERVED. No part of this workbook or manual may be reproduced or transmitted in any form or by any means, electronic or mechanical, including photocopying, or by any information storage or retrieval system, without permission in writing from the publisher.
Manufactured in the United States of America on acid-free paper

04 03 02 01   4 3 2 1

First Edition
American Psychiatric Press, Inc.
1400 K Street, N.W.
Washington, DC 20005
www.appi.org

Adolescent Substance Abuse Intervention Workbook: Taking a First Step ISBN 1-58562-006-8

Staff Manual for Adolescent Intervention Workbook: Taking a First Step ISBN 1-58562-018-1

Staff Manual for Adolescent Substance Abuse Intervention Workbook

Taking a First Step

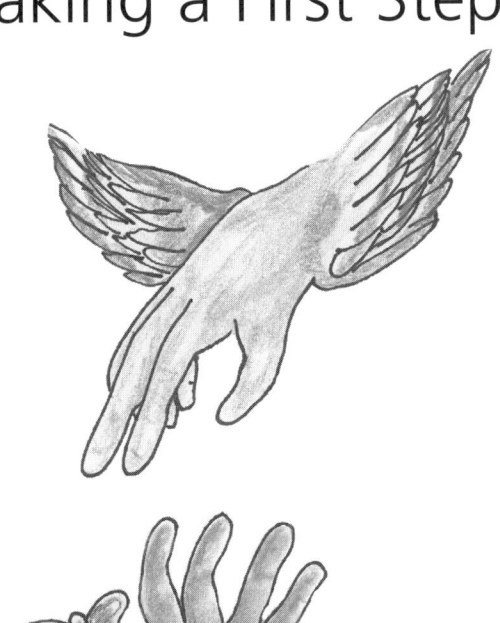

Development of the Adolescent Substance Abuse Intervention Workbook

Drug abuse continues to occur in epidemic proportions in our adolescent population. Efforts need to be made to develop helpful therapeutic tools for assisting teenagers with this problem. In 1990 I published *The Step Workbook For Adolescent Chemical Dependency Recovery: A Guide To The First Five Steps*, which was developed to help teenagers begin to face their drug problems, determine whether they are addicts or are on the way to becoming addicts, and begin to work the steps of a 12-step program (Jaffe 1990).

The steps were placed into a context that would be meaningful for adolescents from a developmental, emotional, and cognitive perspective. Psychiatric issues such as depression, abuse, and learning disabilities were addressed, and psychodynamic, cognitive-behavioral, family, and 12-step approaches were included. This earlier workbook was well received by the treatment community and was used in many inpatient and outpatient programs, probation groups, and outpatient offices. At that time, the length of stay in treatment programs was much longer; treatment staff would spend a week or two developing a relationship with the teenager and then begin encouraging him or her to begin writing a "First Step."

The "First Step" in the five-step workbook comprised many open-ended questions that the patient would answer in phrases or sentences. With the decreasing availability of programs and time for treatment, I recognized that a new workbook suitable for initial treatment of substance-abusing teenagers was needed. This new "First Step" intervention workbook is intended for teenagers who are known to be using some drugs and/or alcohol, but the amounts, frequency, and negative consequences are unrecognized.

The *Adolescent Substance Abuse Intervention Workbook* does not replace the "First Step" in the five-step workbook but is rather an initial tool to help the patient examine his or her drug and/or alcohol use and the associated consequences; after the intervention workbook has been completed, the more open-ended, less structured five-step workbook can be used. The intervention workbook asks concrete, specific questions related to the various consequences of drug and alcohol use. Teenagers do not have to think too much about the questions; they simply circle YES or NO or fill in the blanks. One unique feature of the intervention workbook is the inclusion of *using teen thoughts*—thoughts favoring drug and alcohol use that exist in many of these teenagers but are rarely, if ever, revealed to us—and the contrasting healthy, positive, *recovery teen thoughts* that (we hope) coexist with the using thoughts. I have found that by showing teenagers that we are aware of their using thoughts, we can lower their defensiveness and enhance our connection with them; the workbook includes sample using thoughts and recovery thoughts for this purpose.

The intervention workbook has been developed over the past 3 years using feedback from patients, staff, and mental health professionals. The general feedback I have received from many teenagers in hospital, outpatient, and office treatment programs is that the *Adolescent Substance Abuse Intervention Workbook* is helpful and that the comparison of "Using Teen Thinking" with "Recovery Teen Thinking" is amusing. The workbook is intended as a tool to enhance the therapeutic process, and its effectiveness depends on the skills of the mental health professional. This manual presents my understanding and clinical experiences of some ways to use the workbook effectively.

Theoretical Basis for the Intervention Workbook

Transtheoretical Model

The *Adolescent Substance Abuse Intervention Workbook* can be understood from three frames of reference. The first framework is based on the transtheoretical model of change developed by Prochaska and DiClemente (1982). This framework describes the process of changing addictive behavior by moving through specific stages. In the first stage, called *precontemplation,* the patient is not even thinking of changing his or her behavior. In the second stage, *contemplation,* the patient experiences ambivalence about changing his or her behavior, shifting back and forth between thoughts and feelings in favor of changing the behavior and those opposed to changing the behavior. After contemplation is the third stage, *determination,* in which the patient decides to change, followed by the fourth stage, *action,* in which the changes are actually made. In the fifth and final stage, *maintenance,* the patient continues (maintains) the changed behavior.

Within this framework, the therapist's objective is to help the patient progress toward changing the addictive behavior. This nonconfrontational approach is called *motivational interviewing.* The task of the therapist varies with the patient's stage of thought. The therapist whose patient is in the precontemplation stage should obtain information and present feedback to help the patient become aware of his or her substance abuse problem. For a patient at the contemplation stage, the therapist's motivational task involves helping the ambivalent patient tip the balance toward reasons and feelings that favor change and away from those opposed to change. This framework has been used mainly with adults to help them stop smoking, and little work has been done in using this framework to treat adolescent substance abuse. In applying the stages of change framework to adolescent alcohol and drug abuse, it appears that most adolescents are at either the precontemplation stage or the beginning of the contemplation stage.

DiClemente (1991) describes four types of precontemplators: 1) reluctant (the patient simply lacks knowledge that he or she has a problem); 2) rebellious (the patient resents being told what to do and strenuously resists the thought that he or she may need to change); 3) resigned (the patient feels hopeless and has given up on the possibility of change); and 4) rationalizing (the patient has all the reasons why he or she should not change and why his or her substance abuse is not a problem). To these four types of precontemplators, I would add the restricted-thinking precontemplator. These patients still have active drugs or alcohol in their brains, which prevents them from even thinking about whether they need to change. Because the THC in marijuana is fat soluble and may last from 2 to 3 weeks in brain cells, the precontemplator who uses marijuana heavily will have restricted thinking for several weeks after he or she has stopped using marijuana. In addition, because marijuana causes short-term memory loss, the patient will have difficulty remembering any of what was discussed with the therapist.

A sixth and extremely important type of precontemplator is the faking contemplation patient, which is more prevalent in the adolescent population. Faking contemplation adolescents will discuss the need to stop using and the negative consequences of using, but while telling the therapist the reasons why they should stop using, as is characteristic of the contemplative stage, they are really thinking, "I should just tell these people what they want to hear so I can go back to what I love, which is using drugs and alcohol." Faking contemplation adolescents pretend that they are ambivalent when in actuality they are at the precontemplative stage—they are not truly considering abstaining from the use of drugs and alcohol, they are only pretending to do so. My clinical experience has been that most adolescents exhibit characteristics of the rebellious, rationalizing, and faking contemplation types.

The intervention workbook is designed to help the precontemplative adolescent progress into the contemplative stage. Through writing, discussing, and presenting the workbook answers, reluctant precontemplators will learn of their need to stop using drugs and/or alcohol. Rebellious precontemplators will examine, in a nonconfrontational manner, the negative consequences of their substance abuse and will be presented with a choice of whether to stop using. For resigned precontemplators, the workbook emphasizes that stopping the use of drugs and/or alcohol will give them the power to have a good life. Rationalizing precontemplators, by remembering details of the negative consequences of their substance abuse, will realize how bad their life has become. For restrictive-thinking patients, the simplicity of filling the blanks or circling YES or NO in very concrete answers will help them examine their drug and/or alcohol use despite their limited, reflective thinking.

This workbook is especially helpful for the faking contemplation precontemplator. The "Using Teen Thinking" described earlier is spelled out and contrasted with "Recovery Teen Thinking." Thus, the workbook is used to help move the precontemplative teenager into the contemplative stage of change and help the teenager who is at the contemplative stage to define, in a concrete and personal way, the negative consequences of his or her alcohol and/or drug use. Doing so will help the patient tip the scale of ambivalence toward deciding to change and then progress into the action stage.

12-Step Programs

The second frame of reference is derived from 12-step programs. In this frame of reference, the first step involves admitting that one is powerless over drugs and alcohol and that life has become unmanageable. The intervention workbook helps adolescents examine each area of their lives, identify the negative consequences that have ensued from their use of drugs and/or alcohol, and realize how drugs and alcohol have made life unmanageable. Because the word *powerless* makes teenagers cringe, this word is not used in the workbook. Rather, the emphasis is on the idea that getting off drugs and alcohol will enhance their power. This is especially important for adolescents who have suffered from emotional, sexual, and/or physical abuse. In the intervention workbook, the teenager admits that drugs and/or alcohol have messed up his or her life and that stopping will enhance his or her power.

Psychodynamic Psychiatry

The third frame of reference for the intervention workbook is that of psychodynamic psychiatry. Within this framework, the workbook's "First Step" describes an ego split: the adolescent is shown that he or she has two parts—a using part that communicates drug-using thoughts and a healthy part that is in touch with reality and helps him or her look at long-range goals and not just short-term pleasures. The "Using Teen Thinking" and "Recovery Teen Thinking" illustrated within the workbook are concrete examples of this ego split. Patients are told that their "healthy parts" fill out the workbook, look at their lives, and want positive things to happen. Thus, the intervention workbook helps teenagers become more honest about the extent of their drug and/or alcohol use and the negative consequences that have resulted from it.

Completing the workbook and presenting their answers in a group will also help adolescents undo their ego defense of *disavowal*, a mechanism by which they acknowledge the content of what has happened but deny the emotional meaning of these events. Presenting specific details of drug and/or alcohol use and the negative consequences associated with it evokes memories of these events—the teenager who admits that many bad things have happened, such as being arrested, beaten up, or raped, but states that this was no big deal will undo his or her disavowal by remembering all the details of the event. This recall allows patients to experience negative affect—it permits teenagers to feel the pain and sadness related to their experiences that were avoided at the time because they were drunk or high. The teenager is then able, it is hoped, to realize that life was miserable while he or she was using drugs and alcohol.

Suggestions for Using the Workbook

Clinicians who work with adolescents are well aware that teenagers who use drugs and/or alcohol often lie and minimize their drug use. The intervention workbook, as stated previously, is intended for teenagers who are known to be using some drugs and/or alcohol but at unknown frequency, in unknown quantities, and with unknown consequences. The teenager should be given the workbook with instructions to answer all of the questions honestly. After the teenager answers the questions, which can be done in less than 1 hour, the clinician should review the responses with the teenager and point out places that need elaboration or should be redone in a more honest way. If this review is done on an individual basis in the therapist's office, the therapist can review all of the questions in detail by asking the questions directly to the teenager. The teenager should add to the workbook any corrections and additional information discussed with the therapist during review. I often tell patients that the workbook is like looking in a mirror: it is a tool by which they can examine themselves in an honest way and decide whether they need to make any changes. After individual review, if the teenager is in an outpatient, day-patient, or inpatient program, he or she presents their completed workbook at a substance abuse group meeting. Allowing the teenager to schedule when he or she will present the workbook adds a certain amount of importance and ritual to the process.

At the group meeting, the presenting teenager gives the workbook to another teenager. The teenage group members take turns asking questions from a page in the workbook, and the presenting teenager verbally states his or her answers. These verbal answers are checked by the other group members to see if they correspond to the patient's prior written answers. This review allows the presentation to be a time of additional questions, clarification, and further exploration of important issues. It also fosters feedback from both the staff and the other teenage group members; questions and comments of other teens are often the most pertinent and meaningful to the presenting patient.

The clinical judgment and therapy skills of the staff are critical to the progress of the presentation. The teenager asking the questions should also read the "Using Teen Thinking" and "Recovery Teen Thinking" statements in humorous different voices. If the presenting teenager does not appear to be taking the presentation seriously, the staff leader can intervene and terminate the presentation. The teenager is instructed to present at another group when he or she can be more serious.

At the end of the presentation, the group leader should ask for comments from the group as to whether the patient's intervention workbook has been done honestly. If the group finds that the patient has not answered honestly, they may recommend that the workbook be redone. On the other hand, if the group members find that the patient has answered the questions honestly, they may clap and congratulate the patient on reaching a significant milestone in his or her path to recovery.

Elements of the Workbook

The following are clarifications and specific comments for each section of the workbook.

Section I: Introduction

IA: A Note for the Teenager, p. 9 The emphasis of this note is that teenagers should complete the workbook for themselves so they can decide whether they need to make changes.

IB: Drugs That You Have Used, p. 10 Section IB is a brief outline in which teenagers check off the types of drugs and/or alcohol they have used and the age at which they started using the drug/alcohol. This information is important because the earlier the drug use started, the more severe the patient's problem will be. The drugs are listed in the most frequent order of use; teenagers typically progress along a specific order of drug use, usually starting with cigarettes, beer, and wine and then moving on to marijuana. Problem drinking comes next, and if they continue to progress they may use pills, including uppers and downers, hallucinogens, PCP, ecstasy, cocaine, and heroin. Inhalants, including glue, gas, freon, butane, and white-out, are most commonly used in the eighth grade (early adolescence). The common street names of the drugs are placed in parentheses.

The teenager should also indicate the frequency with which these drugs/drinks have been used over the past 6 months—every month, every week, or every day. When discussing this section with the patient, the therapist should explore an estimate of the amounts consumed. Unlike adult drug abusers and addicts, teenagers use multiple drugs. As they progress from one drug to another they continue to use the earlier drugs as well. Thus, a teenager using LSD and cocaine may also be drinking alcohol, smoking marijuana, and taking pills. The therapist must ask about each of these drugs individually because, in most cases, if one does not ask, the teenager does not tell.

IC: Mixed Thinking, p. 11 The "Mixed Thinking" section introduces the ego split between using thoughts and recovery thoughts described earlier. This also introduces teenagers to the concept of ambivalence—that part of them has thoughts of wanting to use drugs and alcohol and that another part, which develops further as they write and process the workbook, realizes the negative consequences and problems associated with their substance use. This developing recognition of negative consequences enhances their movement into and through the contemplation stage.

Section II: Effects of Drugs and/or Alcohol on Areas of Your Life

Section II examines 12 specific areas of the teenager's life and the consequences of his or her drug and alcohol use on these areas.

II-A: Putting Your Life in Danger, p. 12   This section shows the teenager how drugs and alcohol endanger his or her life. The most common situations for alcohol- and drug-abusing teenagers, such as driving a car while drunk or high, being a passenger in a car whose driver is drunk or high, and engaging in high-risk sexual relationships, are questioned. The teenager must provide specific details of his or her behavior (e.g., how many times, the distance traveled), which helps bring back memories of the things he or she has done. Thus, the teenager who describes driving a car 10 times for an average of 5 miles while high or drunk begins to remember those events. As mentioned earlier, this recall evokes negative affect, which helps the teenager realize, in a personal way, how dangerous his or her behavior has been. The negative emotions associated with the behavior that were avoided previously because the patient was drunk or high are felt for the first time.

The workbook makes use of statements such as "It only takes one accident to kill yourself or someone else" and "It only takes one time to get a disease like AIDS" in this section to remind the teenager that recreational users under the influence are just as capable of endangering themselves or others as addicts. Illustrations show how "Using Teen Thinking" tells teens to lie about their experiences so that they can return to using, whereas the "Recovery Teen Thinking" tells them to be honest because these events are life threatening.

II-B: Putting the Lives of Others in Danger, p. 15   Section II-B shows how the patient's substance abuse puts other people in danger. Specific details about the patient's behavior while using are again reviewed for the purpose of bringing back memories and evoking negative affect. The teenager must face the fact that each time he or she drove a car while high or drunk the lives of each person in that car were put in danger. Other behaviors, such as fighting, threatening others, robbing another person ("hold-up"), buying or selling drugs, and carrying a weapon, are also questioned.

II-C: Increasing Depression, p. 17   In Section II-C the possible relationship between drugs and alcohol and depression is examined. In many teens, depression came first and the use of drugs and/or alcohol became a means of escaping the depression. In other teenagers the drug and/or alcohol use came first, and the depression developed later. In approximately one-third of depressed, substance-abusing teenagers, the substance abuse and depression developed simultaneously. No matter which started first, however, depression is almost always made more severe by drug use. Because no drug lasts forever, the teenager always comes down from the drug high, which makes the depression worse.

II-D: Thinking Less of Yourself, p. 19   Section II-D demonstrates the effects of drugs and alcohol on the teenager's sense of self-worth. Here, teenagers answer questions about whether they did things while using that they had previously thought they would never do.

II-E: Breaking the Law, p. 20   This section relates the use of drugs and alcohol to legal problems. Positive responses to the checklist should be explored in more detail when reviewing the answers or during group presentation. Illustrations show how "Recovery Teen Thinking" emphasizes that being honest helps one become stronger and more powerful.

II-F: Effects on Schoolwork, p. 22   Section II-F contains questions related to the effects that using drugs and/or alcohol has had on the patient's schoolwork and activities. Because of the high incidence of attention-deficit/hyperactivity disorder (ADHD) and learning disabilities (20%–30%) within the substance-abusing adolescent population, many teenagers will have struggled with schoolwork prior to their alcohol and drug use. The issue that these substance-abusing adolescents must understand is that they cannot receive treatment for their ADHD or other learning disorders and thus cannot improve their school-type functioning (e.g., passing high school equivalency tests) if they continue using alcohol and/or drugs.

II-G: Losing the Trust of Your Family, p. 25   Section II-G examines the effects that using drugs and/or alcohol has had on the teenager's relationship to his or her family. Issues such as lying, sneaking out, having a negative attitude, arguing, and giving drugs and/or alcohol to a family member are covered.

II-H: Effects on Your Body and Brain, p. 27   The effects of drugs and alcohol on the teenager's body and brain are reviewed in Section II-H. Memory problems, which especially occur with marijuana use, are evaluated. Marijuana's effects include decreased short-term memory, decreased concentration, and decreased motivation. Hallucinogens may produce flashbacks, and alcohol abuse may cause blackouts.

II-I: Running Away from Painful Feelings, p. 28   Section II-I covers how the teenager uses the effects of drugs and alcohol to escape painful emotions and feelings. The teenager realizes that he or she has used drugs and alcohol to block painful feelings and memories. These memories and feelings can be explored further when the workbook is reviewed individually or presented to a group. Illustrations in this section show how "Recovery Teen Thinking" emphasizes that one has to remember in order to forget—one must remember the bad feelings and memories in order to master them—and that these feelings and memories went away only temporarily while using drugs. Many of these teenagers have histories of sexual and/or physical abuse in their childhoods, and some of these issues may be discussed here.

II-J: Effects on Your Mind, p. 29   The effects of drugs and alcohol on the teenager's mind are examined in Section II-J. Questions relate to various activities that the patient did not do or forgot to do because of his or her alcohol or drug use. These activities include attending school, doing homework, playing sports, attending appointments, and even participating in a family event or date. "Using Teen Thinking" is shown as a rationalization—"I didn't want to do those things anyway"—whereas "Recovery Teen Thinking" looks at the situation honestly—"you paid a price for using."

II-K: Effects on Ability to Control Substance Use, p. 31   Section II-K questions the attempts that the teenager has made to control his or her substance abuse, either by cutting down the amount used or frequency of use or by switching to a different drug (e.g., it is permissible to smoke marijuana as long as they are not doing cocaine). Inability to moderate or control alcohol and/or drug use is an essential feature in making the diagnosis of substance dependency disorder. Question 6 in this section relates to why adolescents relapse. Studies show that the most frequent cause of relapse is being around peers who are drinking and/or using drugs. In this situation, even if the recovering teenager is trying not to use, the exposure to drugs and alcohol becomes too tempting to resist. The next reason for relapse involves the presence of dual disorders, especially depression. In addition, many teenagers relapse because they think they can use drugs or alcohol again but this time without any consequences.

Section II-L: Effects on Plans and Goals for the Future, p. 33   This section explores how drugs and alcohol have affected the teenager's future.

Section III: Summary of Effects

The third section of the workbook allows adolescents to add up the number of areas in their life that their drug and/or alcohol use is destroying. The workbook recognizes that although drugs are fun, the teenager needs to stop using to make his or her life better. The "Using Teen Thinking" illustration that says, "You win this one, but I'll be back" is intended to show patients that using and recovery thoughts and feelings will coexist within them and that they will struggle with issues of relapse throughout their recovery. The choice becomes whether the teenager will do what he or she wants to do—use drugs—or what he or she needs to do, which is stop using.

Section IV: Making a Decision

Section IV shows the teenager that he or she can move from contemplation into determination and thus make a conscious decision to stop using drugs and/or alcohol. Although completing the intervention workbook is a very serious procedure, a touch of humor and having fun while processing the questions is an integral part.

Conclusion

Successful completion of the intervention workbook demonstrates a concrete measure of therapeutic progress that can be documented in progress notes. Although I am presently attempting to evaluate the effectiveness of the workbook, this needs to be examined further through empirical research and comparative treatment studies. An adolescent may not abstain from using drugs and/or alcohol after completing the intervention workbook, but he or she has at least been exposed to the consequences that drug and/or alcohol use have had on his or her life. My hope is that at a later time these teenagers will be willing to do what is needed to make their lives better.

Successful completion of the intervention workbook should lead to further treatment. This may include individual and family counseling, after-care groups, 12-step treatment (e.g., meetings, sponsorships, developing a recovering peer group), cognitive-behavioral skill development, and psychiatric treatment of comorbid disorders.

References

DiClemente CC: Motivational interviewing: the stages of change, in Motivational Interviewing. Edited by Miller WR, Rollnick S. New York, Guilford, 1991, pp 191–202

Jaffe SL: The Step Workbook for Adolescent Chemical Dependency Recovery. Washington, DC, American Psychiatric Press, 1990

Prochaska JO, DiClemente CC: Transtheoretical therapy: toward a more integrated model of change. Psychotherapy Theory, Research, and Practice 19:276–288, 1982

Suggested Reading

American Academy of Child and Adolescent Psychiatry: Practice parameters for the assessment and treatment of children and adolescents with substance use disorders. J Am Acad Child Adolesc Psychiatry 36(suppl):140S–156S, 1997

Bukstein OG: Adolescent Substance Abuse. New York, John Wiley & Sons, 1995

Jaffe SL (guest editor): Adolescent substance abuse and dual disorders. Child and Adolescent Psychiatric Clinics of North America 5:1–261, 1996

Kaminer Y: Adolescent Substance Abuse. New York, Plenum Medical, 1994